POLIO'S
PLAYGROUND

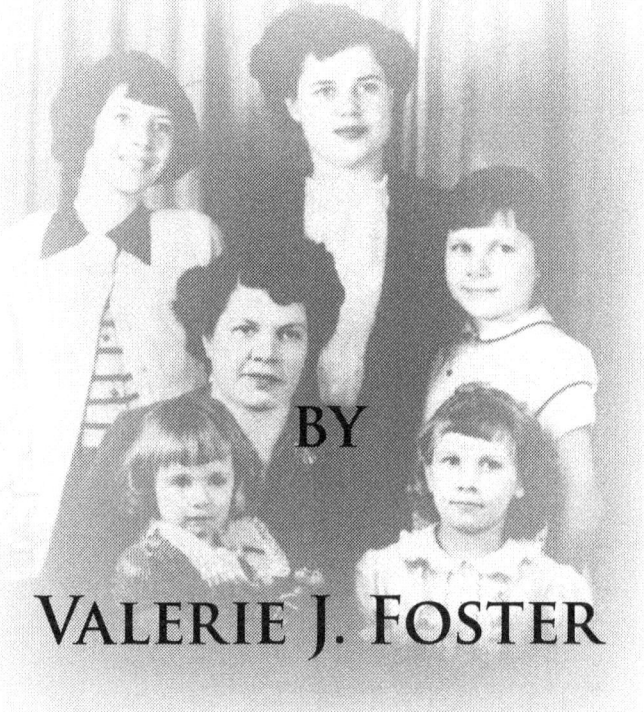

BY

VALERIE J. FOSTER

authorHOUSE™

1663 LIBERTY DRIVE, SUITE 200
BLOOMINGTON, INDIANA 47403
(800) 839-8640
WWW.AUTHORHOUSE.COM

AuthorHouse™
1663 Liberty Drive, Suite 200
Bloomington, IN 47403
www.authorhouse.com
Phone: 1-800-839-8640

AuthorHouse™ UK Ltd.
500 Avebury Boulevard
Central Milton Keynes, MK9 2BE
www.authorhouse.co.uk
Phone: 08001974150

First published by AuthorHouse   2/10/2006

ISBN: 1-4208-8236-8 (sc)

Printed in the United States of America
Bloomington, Indiana

This book is printed on acid-free paper.

Forward

Valerie Foster should have "Doctor," which means "teacher," in front of her name, for she passionately teaches each reader's hearty and soul through her journey with poliomyelitis.

At the heart of this woman's experience is a preventable disease which has ravaged millions of people throughout the world. Realize, at the same time, that wee within a year or two of eradicating this scourge from our planet.

At the soul of this story are courage, hope, and a duty to persevere. This story is a life long representation of these qualities.

Lastly, a reminder to all of us, that respect and kindness, particularly to the vulnerable, is a healing gift in equal measure to our souls and to their challenged spirits. Its absence wounds forever.

Please read on. Travel with Valerie and dare to imagine a world without the disease.

Eric Overland, MD.

June 13, 2004

Acknowledgments

This little book came out of an invitation to speak to the Medford, Oregon Rotary Club about my experience of having poliomyelitis. The rotary clubs across the nation are raising funds to vaccinate the populations in the countries where polio still leads an active life. Thank you Dr. Overland that initial invitation.

Dr. Overland later arranged for an infection disease specialist to review the medical accuracy of my account. And, he has written a gracious forward. Thank-you again.

Tee Corrine is a teacher of writing at Rogue Community College, Grants Pass/Medford, Oregon. I began to write my memoirs when I took her class, "Writing Your Life Story." Thank you, Tee, for all your encouragement, guidance, and your wonderful teaching gift.

Several people heard or read portions of my story and asked me to pursue writing a book. They leant me much support. Thank you Pat, Betty, Ruth, Sierra, and , my sister, Thada.

Tee introduced me to Marilyn Hammer, who owns Jmar Publications. She encouraged me to submit my completed manuscript to her company. Thank you Marilyn for everything you have done to make this book possible. This second edition is being published by AuthorHouse, and I thank them for all their help.

Appreciation and gratefulness is extended to my main editor also; thank you Lorna Romano.

Most of all I want to thank my loving, kind, and supportive husband, Robert Foster. Without his daily support, I would not be who I am today.

CONTENTS

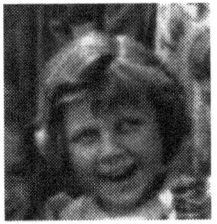

Valerie-Second Grade

POLIO'S PLAYGROUND

PART I: CHILDHOOD PLAYGROUND TO HOSPITALIZATION

I loved going to the Yakima Sportsman Park, outside of Yakima, Washington, where my sisters and I could ride the merry-go-round, sail through the air on the big swings, wade in the pond, and ride the rhythmic see-saw. There lived beautiful peacocks who roamed the grounds freely. I loved it when one would fan his tail in all its glory.

However, the merry-go-round would make me sick to my stomach, so my big sister, Thada, would scold me, "You know it makes you sick; why do you ride it?" I knew inside that it was because I wanted to be just like my big sisters, who loved the merry-go-round. Thada and Charlene, 13¾ and 12 years old respectively, took care of me as I tagged along on our country adventures. I was only eight and had just finished second grade at Moxee Central School, where I was quite a little social butterfly. I received high marks on my school work and the teachers and kids seemed to like me. I loved school, my friends and all of nature. It was the summer of 1952.

Thada, Charlene, and I liked to escape to the park as often as possible in the summer time. Our family was kind of difficult. Mom and Dad fought a lot. Dad would hit Mama around but she had a temper too. She meted out her frustrations in harsh punishment on we girls. So my sisters and I escaped into our creative playtime of fun excursions. One time Thada and Charlene created a "club," and I was the initiate. I had to cross the railroad bridge and knock on "Old man Mac's" door. Then once I did everything they said, the "club" disbanded.

Another fond memory was on "Blackberry Island." It was actually a little island in the middle of the Yakima River's run off tributary that ran along the west and south border of our sixteen acre farm. We pretended that we were homeless orphans and had to live off the land. The only way you could access the island was to walk the barbed wire fence that separated the properties. The creek had quite a current there, so crossing it seemed really hazardous, according to my eight year old mind. But it was worth it because the blackberries were delicious.

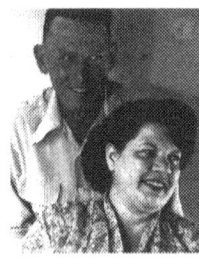
Charles and Juanita Ellison

Those carefree days of summer were prematurely gone that year. On Thursday, June 12, 1952, I was first to get sick with a tremendous headache and a high fever. I was nauseated and weak. Mom thought I had the flu, but on Saturday morning when I screamed that a train was running over my head, she called the family doctor, A.J. Myers, D.O. He came out to our farm, took a look at me, and immediately said that my Mom and Dad needed to take me to the hospital. I went to the little osteopathic hospital in Yakima, where they preformed many diagnostic tests, including a spinal tap for meningitis or poliomyelitis, more commonly known as, polio.

Both tests came back negative. Since both Thada and Charlene became sick in the next few days, they were taken to the largest hospital in the county, St. Elizabeth, where they both tested positive for polio. On June 17, I was given another spinal tap which tested positive this time. They transferred me to St. Elizabeth's Hospital. We were known as "The Ellison Sisters" and we were big news in the *Yakima Herald*, because not even the Yakima City County health officer, Dr. Stanley Brenner, or attending physicians had knowledge of a case where three members of the same family were stricken at the same time.

One of the worst national epidemics of polio was experienced across the United States that year; the number of victims reached an unprecedented 57,628. Children were dropping like flies—coming down with the disease—sometimes dying from bulbar polio, which affects the brain, but also from the other two types: spinal and respiratory. If they didn't die, they were usually, but not always, left with the crippling effects of this virus.

In the 1920's, 90% of the cases of polio were in children under the age of five, thus it was called "infantile paralysis." In the early 20th century there were police squads that would scour the streets looking for children who were sick. They were trying to arrest the spread of the disease, so they would take the children away from their parents to hospitalize them because the kids were suspected of harboring the virus. Although only one case in a thousand causes permanent paralysis, parents were afraid of the crippling menace. Our story was in the news paper every few days..

Three Sisters Stricken With Polio Attack

Three of four sisters in one Yakima family are the first victims of polio in Yakima County this year. Daughters of Mr. and Mrs. Charles Ellison, 405 Keys Rd., the three girls are in St. Elizabeth Hospital for treatment.

The girls are Valerie, 8; Charlene, 12, and Thada, 14. Their sister Kathie 4, has thus far escaped the disease.

Attending physicians had not personally known of a case where three members of the same family were stricken at the same time, nor had Dr. Stanley Benner, Yakima City-County health officer. Records show, however, that such cases have existed, they said.

Valerie First

Valerie, who has some involvement of her chest and both arms, was the first to develop polio symptoms. She complained she was not feeling well last Friday morning, her mother said, and was kept home from church school. Her main complaint was a headache.

Doctors were called and on Sunday she was taken to the hospital for tests, which were inconclusive. Back home, the child seemed better until Tuesday, when the other two girls, Charlene and Thada began showing symtoms of polio. All three were hospitalized in the isolation ward and polio was confirmed, attending physicians said.

In Iron Lung

Charlene, was perhaps the hardest hit and is in an iron lung which assists her in breathing.

Thada, has some involvement in both her legs. All are in good spirits and have shown much improvement since Wednesday, doctors said.

Fifteen cases of polio were confirmed during 1951, according to Dr. Benner. The first was in March and the last on December 10. October was the high month, with a total of five.

6-20-52

Polio changed everyone's life, especially my family's. People were afraid to let their children go swimming, or even play with neighborhood friends. Although polio is contagious only for the initial two to three weeks, no one wanted their child exposed to the risk of this crippling disease. So I never saw my friends again. This was one of my more difficult adjustments. This made for a very isolating experience for an eight year old. But I had my sisters. We were the first cases of the "polio season" that year. Even the Associated Press Institute (API) picked up our story for the national news.

Other than that headache, like a train-running-over-my-head, the first spinal tap was one of the things I clearly remember. It involves a syringe that the doctor uses to draw fluid from around the spinal column. The nurses and my Mom held me in a tight fetal position while the doctor stuck the needle in the small of my back. I screamed bloody murder and tried to get loose, but they held me tight. Since the test came out negative they pumped me full of penicillin, injecting me every three hours, until my bottom felt like a pin cushion. The nurses coaxed, coerced, or bribed me into drinking lots of water and Koolaid, while the doctors puzzled over what was making me so sick. That Tuesday morning, after the second spinal tap, during which I was too weak to put up much resistance, and before I went to St. Elizabeth's, I asked Mom to scratch my head because I couldn't raise my right arm and the other arm was strapped to an intravenous (IV) tube. Paralysis was setting in. Dr. Meyers did not have privileges at St. Elizabeth's Hospital therefore we would need to be under the care of another doctor. So we all three were placed in the same isolation ward.

During the contagious, isolation phase of polio, the nasty little virus bugs eat away at specific nerve cells in the brain and spinal column. These are the nerves that send messages to the muscles. If those cells are damaged or killed, the muscles are compromised or completely paralyzed. 95% of polio cases are unrecognized or are so mild that they don't cause any symptoms. It doesn't happen with the snap of your fingers but can take up to 19 days for paralysis to set in. For both Charlene and I, paralysis was from the neck down. Thada's legs were paralyzed but she appeared to have no involvement from the waist up.

The public outcry for a vaccine resounded throughout the nation. Scientists were working around the clock. The development of an inoculation turned into an interesting political and economical battle between backers of both Dr. Jonas Salk and Dr, Albert Sabin. Dr. Salk's "inactivated virus" was used in trial runs before its release for public use in 1955. Americans were overjoyed that we at last had a method of prevention. Salk killed the virus before developing the vaccine. So if you were inoculated by his method, contagion was not a risk factor. The preventative dose was administered by injection and it was believed to require three "booster" shots. It was costly to distribute and store. But it was available and it did provide protection from the dreaded disease. We three girls, as well as our two younger sisters, did receive the Salk shots when they were available in 1955, because we had contracted only two types of polio, spinal and respiratory. The vaccination provided immunity for all three kinds of polio, including bulbar, which we had not caught. There were also trial runs of Sabin's vaccine, it was released to the public in oral form in 1962. It was not only administered orally, which was less objectionable, but it held life long immunity and it was much easier, and cost effective, to distribute and store.

The treatments for recovery were like a playground where you could run from one apparatus to another, such as merry-go-round to swings, to jungle gym, to teeter-totter. Initially, as I said, I was paralyzed from the neck down, but I rapidly regained use of many muscles through therapies: physical therapy, hydrotherapy, and hot-pack treatment. The experience of the hot pack remedy was among the worst. Wool, double-folded "blankets," about the size of a small bath towel, and smelling of pungent disinfectant, were soaked in a boiling solution, wrung out in a special bucket, then flopped onto our inert, exposed skin of our various body parts: legs, arms, back, stomach, neck and chest. If the nurse was compassionate, she might fan them twice in the air to reduce the heat a little. But if the nurse was tired, frustrated, and/or impatient, she might shake it once to straighten it out from the wringer, and slap it on. One day Charlene's arm was burnt by a hot-pack. She hollered out. She was unable to get it off because of her paralysis, but the nurse just left it, perhaps not realizing that it was actually burning her arm. Of course the staff treated the burn but did not reveal it to the doctor. Things like that didn't happen often, most of the time the nurses were kind and caring. It just seems like the bad times stick a little harder in my memory.

Hydrotherapy had a component similar to the Sportsmen's Park in that the water was soothing, but it was also scary. After changing me into these flimsy bikini-type-tie-on panties, Charlene got a bra too, the therapists would lift me into a sling that would sway over the hydrotherapy pool. This was a communal pool, where many children would receive treatment. Then I would be slowly, or not so slowly, lowered into the 102° water. The sling would be removed, leaving me floating. The procedure was extremely frightening for me and very embarrassing for my older sisters because they were scantily clad in this communal pool. I was totally vulnerable because I had no way to protect myself. When I was afloat, someone had to be close at hand because my body might begin to roll and I could not turn my head to keep my mouth and nose out of water. I was at the complete mercy of my nurses and therapists. Although I felt vulnerable, the warm water was ever so soothing. While in the water, a physical therapist would move my legs, arms, fingers, and toes. Every muscle she had been taught to identify was flexed and exercised.

Besides the "hot-pack" treatment and the hydrotherapy, we also "played" physical therapy. I dreaded it as did most of the children. Some of the therapists were likeable, but others were just plain mean. When we were paralyzed and lying in one place, our muscles would tighten. They needed to be stretched and flexed. Remember there is no damage to the actual muscle; the damage is to the nerves that send the messages to the muscles. Therefore the muscles lie dormant and are paralyzed. To keep the muscles healthy, and to promote as much nerve healing as possible, physical therapy was a daily activity. This torture was meted out by both the "likeable" and the "mean" therapists, who definitely had different approaches.

Physical therapy started once we were past the contagious and feverish stage. The therapist would move my leg in every direction a leg is suppose to move. She would stretch the muscles as far as possible, pushing hard to get maximum pull on the muscle. For instance, my therapist would lift my leg straight off the bed, keeping it straight with her arm. She would be up on the bed, on her knees, and lean her body forward into my leg, pushing it as far toward my head as she could. Now, as an adult, I understand what they were doing in the name of medicine, but as a child, this whole procedure seemed highly unnecessary. Another exercise was to bend my ankle up toward my shin to loosen the tendons down the back of my ankle. It was particularly painful. This had the potential for someone to work out their hostilities toward children, and I firmly believe that some of those therapists had huge anger issues. Besides being overzealous at times, the particularly uncompassionate therapists were also unlikely to give me time to catch my breath, no matter how much I was crying out in pain.

To assist my breathing I was placed in an iron lung. Only my head stuck out from the cylindrical machine. A rubber collar encircled my neck. The sides of the tube had glass "portholes," like a ship. My caretakers could put their hands through the rubber rimmed glass section to examine, tend, and bathe my body. It felt like my body was detached from my head. Although I couldn't feel any air movement, I could feel the pressure that made my lungs deflate and expand. I was only in an iron lung for two days. Another patient needed it worse than I. (The hospital only had two iron lungs. My sister, Charlene, was using one. Without it she would have died.) I was placed on the next polio playground ride: a rocking bed, which was a weird teeter-totter ride.

The rocking bed machine rotated with an autonomic mechanism. The head of the bed would tip down to a 45° angle, and gravity would pull the air from my lungs. Then the foot of the bed would drop down to a 45° angle, stopping the resistance to the air entering my lungs. Although I don't remember exactly how often this would repeat, I know the cycle was several times a minute. This "ride" was nauseating though, like the merry-go-round of earlier days. I remember thinking it was okay because it did help me breathe.

I shared my isolation room with Thada. Charlene was across the hall in her own room because she needed more care. Sometimes Thada would giggle and holler across the hall to her, "Hey Charlene, you still there?" We would hear a faint giggle and her voice respond, "Yeah, I'm here." Things I remember from that isolation room were counting the dots in the acoustical ceiling tiles; learning to feed myself again. They gave me Jell-o that kept falling off my spoon which would make me laugh. Thada and I told stories to each other. I also remember Thada singing camp songs to me, and "The Witch."

"The Witch" was our name for a grouchy, big-nosed nurse with black hair, who attended our care both in isolation and in the big ward. She was rough and always scolding us for some little infraction. By the end of the third week in the hospital I had some movement in my arms. I never did regain the ability to raise my right arm above my head, but my forearm was working okay, enabling me to hold a book or crayons to color. "The Witch" would scold me because I left my crayons on the bed. Or she would complain to Thada that she left her book on the bed instead of putting it on the bedside table. What a grouch! She was also weird. She would give us enemas and then carry the bedpan around showing all the children what a "good job" we had done. It was both embarrassing and gross. I would think that she was the sick one, not me.

After the first weeks, I was no longer "sick." Now that I was breathing better and able to feed myself again, I was placed in a six-bed ward where there were eventually eleven children. Charlene remained in the isolation ward where she could receive more individualized care even though she was no longer contagious. Thada came along with me to the larger ward. There were so many patients that year they were even placed in the hallways.

The big ward, in ways, was like sitting around the campfire in Sportsman Park telling ghost stories. We would talk back and forth telling jokes, riddles, or some story about school or our individual adventures. Thada and the other older girls talked about boys a lot. Our ward consisted of all girls as far as I remember. I don't recall if they had a boy's ward or not. It doesn't seem probable that only girls were hospitalized there, and yet, I seem to remember only the girls. We were from all over the Yakima Valley; various schools and different cities were represented.

Even though we were in the hospital, there were fun times. Most of the happy memories were from the big ward, such as the birthday party for Sylvia Hanson. Charlene was out of the iron lung by then, in the big ward with me, and Thada had been discharged. Charlene could not move her arms and we both had to be carried into our chairs for the festivities. Mrs. Hanson bought all of us party hats, napkins, cups, and little trinkets. We had cake, ice cream and candy. The Yakima Herald reporter came and once again took a picture.

Also in the big ward, I was the storyteller. After lights would be turned off at 8pm, I would tell a story to my ward mates. They were simple little stories, usually about animals, which I called my nature friends.

Sometimes the nurses would scold us to stop giggling and go to sleep, like it was a slumber party.

Before I left the hospital, I had to learn how to walk again. After being placed in a standing position, between the parallel bars, wearing two heavy, metal leg braces, I was directed to walk to the other end, about eight feet. The therapist would be close so she could catch me if I faltered. I remember how hard I had to concentrate to get my leg to move. I was training new nerves to do the job of the damaged nerves. I would literally be sweating after I was able to accomplish this simple task. But for me that wasn't the hardest part of having polio.

Part II: Public Perceptions and Reactions

The hardest part was having my emotional needs ignored. I did not understand what was happening to me. It really was a shame that so many adults didn't give me the right to be included in the decision making process about my own body. Nothing was explained to me; I was just expected to cooperate, which I did most of the time. I was just a little girl who needed to be led into healing this assault to my body, mind and soul. The medical staff were excellent at meeting my body needs. They pretty much ignored my mental and emotional needs.

And, there were plenty of crackpots who would write letters to us or send get-well cards with the message inside that we were being punished for our sins. I struggled to understand how I had sinned to warrant such stringent discipline. One of my most horrendous memories was when we were bringing Charlene home from the hospital after her long stay. She was in a wheelchair. She had never regained use of either arm and her entire body muscles were very compromised. Mother was slowly pushing and I was holding on to the arm of the chair to give me balance. We were still in the parking lot moving towards our car when this woman blocked the chair from progressing. She leaned into Charlene's face. The woman's hands gripped each arm of the chair as she loudly proclaimed, "Repent! Repent my child! For this is God's punishment!" Mother pushed the chair forward and hollered for the woman to get out of the way. The woman stumbled to the side but still yelled, "You have sinned and this is God's way!!" Being eight years old, I was negatively influence by this nonsense. Although for years I pondered my own thoughts and behaviors, I never came to understand that concept of punishment; I had always viewed God as loving.

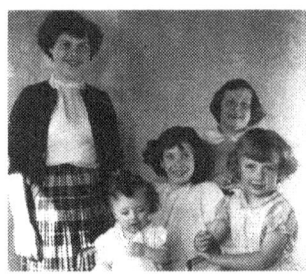

Thada, Rhonda, Charlene, Valerie, & Kathy

I left the hospital after 4½ months, on October 1, 1952. My youngest sister, Rhonda Gail, was born on October 9th. Thada had been home for about a month previous to my release. I took various assistive devices home with me: two leg braces, a back brace, an arm brace, and crutches. In a few months I had worked my way out of the left leg brace, reduced my right leg brace to one that was below my knee, and no longer needed crutches to keep my balance. However we lived in the country and had no indoor plumbing. On January 4th, the day before I was to return to school, I slipped and fell on my way to the outhouse. My right leg was severely broken above my knee. A cast stabilizing my hip, knee, and ankle was necessary. Since this cast encircled my waist and continued all the way down my right side, I was once again bed ridden for another two and a half months. We did get an inside bathroom that year and I finally returned to school in April, right after my ninth birthday.

I no longer went to the country school; I wasn't able to negotiate the Moxee Elementary staircases. I still wore the back brace and for a few months a full right leg brace. My left arm brace and the crutches were history. Mom drove me into town to Hoover Elementary, which had a special education wing and a speech and physical therapy department that included a hydrotherapy pool. Most of my classmates were mentally delayed. The other kids called them the dumbies. Why was I in there? I thought, "I'm not dumb." It was only about a week or so later that they moved me into a regular classroom with a teacher that I will never forget, Mrs. Pengelly.

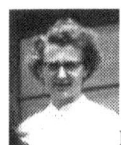
Mrs. Pengelly
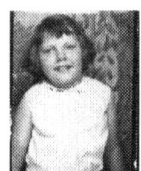
Third Grade

Before going back to school, Mom warned me that the kids might tease me because of my "handicaps." I don't remember any such taunts. However, Mom hadn't said anything about teasing because I was fat. Without much exercise and with added treats, I was looking fairly roly-poly. My last name being Ellison, I was sometimes called "Elephant." And, because I liked to talk a lot, I was also called "Chatty Fatty."

However, Mrs. Pengelly was always looking out for me. She would either distract the other kids, or take me away from such teasing. She would sometimes give me things to do in the classroom, so I wouldn't need to go out to the playground. I felt truly loved by her.

I missed all but two months of my third grade. The school administration allowed me to test out of third grade and I was promoted to fourth grade with my classmates. Fourth, fifth, and sixth grades were filled with the average trials and tribulations of friends, teachers, and family. Mom and Dad's fights escalated. Miss Stapleton in fourth grade accused me of cheating when I really didn't cheat. I never really cared for my fifth grade teacher. And in Mr. Roberts sixth grade class, I would always be the umpire during classroom baseball games. That added to my feelings of isolation from the other kids. But I found one particular friend with whom friendship continued on into junior high school, Joan Roller. We were buds clear through to ninth grade.

After school in the evening, three times a week, the physical therapist would come and pull out the kitchen table, to be used for a therapy platform. The therapist was usually Dan Felthouse, but sometimes was Helen Hazen. They would give all three sisters our treatments.

Besides school and treatments, we still had to do our farm and house chores like any other family. Of course Mom had the worst of it: new baby, taxi service (both Charlene and I needed to go to separate schools in town—and we had therapies and surgeries), farm chores (canning, gardening, cows to milk, pigs to slop, eggs to gather, etc.), laundry, cooking, general childcare, including the special care for Charlene.

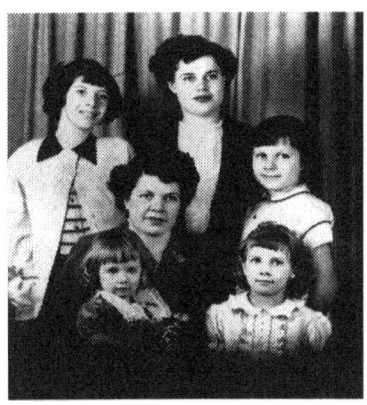

Mom and Her Five Girls 1954

As I grew, the effects of polio's damage took me on a new ride. In 1957, age thirteen, I could not sit unassisted. The full body brace helped, but it was not supporting me adequately. The right muscles of my upper back were stronger than the left side, pulling my spine to the right. Slightly lower the muscle strength was the opposite, pulling my spine to the left. Lower still, it reversed again and in the lumbar region the curvature again changed. This crisscross pattern created an "s" curvature (scoliosis), as well as a forward curving of the spine (kyphosis). The crookedness was becoming so severe I could no longer sit without the brace. In the morning, I would tuck my metal and leather brace under the covers to warm it up. Then I would roll around to get my back into it while I was still lying down. I would close the top section over the top of me and fasten the leather straps. I could then sit up, put my leg brace on and get dressed. Polio was taking me on another ride.

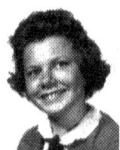
Age 13

It was becoming increasingly painful to sit or stand. The doctors decided I needed a spine fusion. The summer between my seventh and eighth grade was devoted to a couple of surgeries: a fifteen vertebrae spine fusion and a right ankle tendon transplant. The nerves that triggered the muscles to lift my right ankle were dead. So the surgeon would stretch the muscles of my fourth toe, transplanting its function to my ankle, making it possible for me to lift my foot. No more "drop foot."

The Chief of Orthopedics at Children's Hospital in Seattle, Washington, Dr. John Lacocq, would perform the spine fusion. So the week following school closure in June 1957, Mother and I packed up and drove the 250 miles to the other side of the Cascade Mountains. After I was settled in my room, she needed to drive back home again; she could not afford to stay in a motel and my sisters needed her care. It was scary to be alone but I trusted Dr. Lacocq; he was a gentle man.

He explained every detail to me, the only doctor who ever did. For two weeks my spine needed to be stretched out, so it would be perfectly straight and be at its maximum length to get the most benefit for me. This whole process brought me feelings of embarrassment and extreme vulnerability. Children's Hospital was a teaching medical center, so student doctors and nurses would gather around to view the procedures. I would be mortified to have my newly budding breasts exposed for all to see; I was usually dressed in only my panties. Placing me on a double hammock-like bed, an eight pound weight was attached to each of the various harnesses. There was head gear, two shoulder harnesses, a hip attachment, a waist harness, and each foot was tethered. The whole apparatus could be rotated so my face would be up toward the ceiling, or down towards the floor. Therefore they could equally distribute the pull of gravity and minimize the possibilities of bedsores. The "hammocks" had a hole for my face, or it cradled the back of my head. When I was on my back, and it was time to rotate, they would place the front "hammock" on top of me, turn the whole thing over and remove the back half. Later I learned this was called a "Stryker Frame (or Bed)." Although Mother sometimes came to visit me on the weekends, those first two weeks were long and very uncomfortable. But, I grew three inches, the tallest I have ever been, 5'3".

Next, they formed a body cast, which was split

in half down the sides. Using this, I would lie in the shells to maintain my stretched out form. I thought I was probably going to be in this contraption even longer. But it was just one or two mornings later that I was to go to surgery. The nurse woke me up at 5:00 am to give me a shot to relax me. I was nice and calm as they readied me for my eight o'clock operation. No food or drink that morning for me. I was given a full body sponge bath, after which they shaved my back and my right leg. After rubbing a putrid disinfectant on the targeted areas, I was wrapped in a warm, fuzzy, towel-like blanket. At about 6:30, Dr. Nash, Dr. Lacocq's assistant surgeon, came in to place a metal pin into the bone of the ending vertebrae. That way they wouldn't need to count them in the midst of the actual operation. Not knowing what he was going to do, I just cooperated to get into position. But when he placed the pin, about the size of a straight pin, on my back, took a rubber mallet and pounded it, I screamed! The nurse had "forgotten" to give me the local anesthetic. The doctor was furious. He ordered something to be given to me immediately, loudly proclaiming," We cannot reschedule this surgery."

Nothing short of knocking me out was going to make me relax after that experience. I was administered the "Novocain," or whatever it was, and the doctor returned in about a half hour. I could still feel much of what he was doing. I cried or screamed throughout the undertaking. I did not want to hold still. "Heck! I didn't even want to be there. The nurses held me down while the doctor was yelling at both the nurses and me. Finally the pin was in. I was taken to the operating room, put into a diaper (how humiliating), strapped onto a table and IV's were placed in both arms. I truly welcomed going to sleep.

The only thing that Dr. Lacocq had not told me is that this procedure would take two separate days. Dr. Nash was able to finish the tendon transplant on my ankle, but I needed to go back into surgery the next day to finish the spinal part. No more pins though—whew! I was in a lot of pain and did not want further surgery, but it wasn't up to me. Obviously they needed to complete the fusion.

This was more than 45+ years ago; spine fusions were done differently then. The surgeon opened my back the length of the intended fusion. From each side of every nodule of the vertebrae, a slice of bone was removed with a surgical saw, and then placed in the space between the vertebrae. When the bone fused, it would create a solid spine down the length of the procedure. Three of my cervical and twelve of my thoracic vertebrae were fused, for a total of fifteen. Both the fusion and the tendon transplant were very successful for me.

I probably remember that hospital stay in more detail because I was five years older than my initial contact with polio, but I remember it more because of the absolute boredom, John, and one nurse's abusive behavior. I lay there with hours and hours to just think. I was in a room with a girl about my same age. I'm not sure of her name, but I think it was Rosemary. She was born with a facial deformity. To the best of my memory, she was having her seventeenth facial surgery. All procedures were steps to give her a nose and reset her eyes. She was also having a spine fusion the day after mine. My screaming when they had to set the pin, absolutely terrified her. Fortunately, she only needed a couple of vertebrae fused, so they didn't need to mark her spine with a pin. And I felt blessed to not have her facial problems.

I was happy to have John too. He was 12 years old and my good friend who visited me from his room every day. He was an Indian boy who had terminal bone cancer. He was from the White Swan Reservation Orphanage and had no parents, I overheard a nurse say. He was such a positive support for me; he was always happy and would make me laugh. I regret that I did not keep in contact with him.

And then there was that nurse. She was a loud, obnoxious woman. After the surgery, to my surprise, I was placed in a regular bed, not on the Stryker Frame. Lying in my cast shells, the hours would tick away for another month and a half. Volunteers would sometimes come to read to me, and the routine of daily hospital life was soon memorized: wake up at six am, breakfast served at 7:30, right after shift change, and bed bath at 9:00. This monotony was gladly interrupted when Phil Harris and Bing Crosby visited us. However, Bing Crosby was a real grouch that day, and it changed my feelings for him no matter how well he could sing. Phil Harris was real nice. Another time, Gordon Scott, "Tarzan," came to see the children. It was quite exciting.

During this hospital stay, "Nurse Loud" was my regular day nurse three days a week. I dreaded those days. I had begun my menstrual cycles when I was eleven, but with the surgeries, I was irregular, never knowing when "it" would arrive. This particular morning, when she came to give me a bed bath, I told her I thought my period had started. She walked down the hallway loudly saying to all the other nurses, or anyone who could hear her, "Valerie has dyed her hair red, she does it once a month." She soon returned, holding a pair of scissors, clicking them open and shut as she walked, singing, "Valerie's getting a hair cut, Valerie's getting a hair cut."

I truly hated her at that moment. I was shy, humiliated and silent. She needed to clip away some of the clotted blood. Maybe it wasn't sexual abuse in terms of it being sexually gratifying for her, but it was definitely very abusive to my young teenage ego. I was physically in a very vulnerable position and she took the opportunity to capitalize on my vulnerability for her own perverse enjoyment.

The healing from those two surgeries took many more months. To stabilize both my neck and my hips, the cast, upon discharge, was wrapped around my head and extended low on my hips. It also held my left elbow (bent at a 90° angle skyward) in a raised, right angle to my body. I was unable to sit or stand. I would still need a hospital bed, which was placed in our living room. I would lean clear over the side of the bed, with my plate of food on a chair beside the bed, and eat upside down. Mom was very busy and very stressed, often not able to feed me. In addition to keeping care of me, she had the farm duties and my four sisters. By now Rhonnie, the baby, was almost five years old, Kathy was nine, Charlene was seventeen. Thada was nineteen, married and staying with us with her newborn baby, Johnny, while her Navy husband was "out to sea."

Keep in mind that Charlene needed much care. She was extremely thin and most of the muscles throughout her body were atrophied. At 5'1" tall she weighed 65 lbs. She never regained use of her arms. She only had a little movement in her left hand. She had learned to prop her arm on the table edge, hold a fork precariously, and with leverage move her arm towards her mouth. Then she would bend down and retrieve her food from the fork. She could paint pictures with her toes, and she could type with a pencil in her mouth. She was able to sign her name with her hand in the same manner as she fed herself. All of these feats were very difficult and sapped her energy. Charlene also had very weak lung muscles and had spent two and a half months in an iron lung. She had trouble coughing up mucus when she had a cold. Many times I helped Charlene hang upside down over the edge of her bed, pounding on her back to dislodge and release the phlegm. Mom tried to protect her, but each year she would catch at least one cold, if not two, that would send her to the hospital with pneumonia. 1957 would be the last year she had to endure those hospitalizations.

By October of that year, my hospital bed was returned. In the morning, either Mom or Dad would carry me from my bedroom to the living room, and vice versa at night. I must have been a hefty load; I wore the plaster-of-Paris full body cast. By then, the cast on my right lower leg, from the transplant, had been reduced to an ace bandage wrap. Mom cut a baby mattress into two parts and covered them separately with brown corduroy to be used as floor cushions. During the day, I could lay on the cushions in the living room and be among the family activity, watching TV, playing cards, etc. Come bedtime, I would be carried back to the bedroom.

October 1st was the day I went home from the hospital after initially contracting polio in 1952. Exactly five years later, on October 1st, 1957, Charlene died. This time the pneumonia took her. She weighed only 45 lbs. at the time of her death. This was a great loss for everyone who knew her. The previous year, the local Altrusa Club had elected Charlene as "Girl of the Year." She conducted guest sermons at our Baptist Church and received a straight "A" average in her academic work. She always smiled and had an encouraging word for others. It was a HUGE loss for me; she was my best friend and confidant.

I couldn't attend her funeral because I was still

in this very restrictive body cast. In my young mind's grieving, I would see her in heaven reaching across the family dinner table for a slice of bread, something she could not do in actual life. She was "whole" again. But I was still on polio's playground, so I took a deep breath and continued on with my life.

Each month I would return to Children's hospital to have x-rays and the cast modified. The first alteration was to raise the front bottom of the cast so that I could bend my hips to a sitting position. The next month they set my lower left forearm free. The elbow was still extended out at a 90° angle from my body.

In a few more months, the doctor ordered more of the bottom cut away, removed the arm extension, and lowered the cast behind my head. It didn't let all my hair fall free, but the top half of my hair could fall over the cast now. Each modification gave me slightly more movement. By February 1958, when I started back to school, I was in a new back brace. This one was similar to the cast shells I had lain in right after the fusion. It hinged on the right side and was shaped like a sleeveless, scoop-neck blouse in the front. It had a high back that didn't dip down like a blouse but didn't extend up the back of my head. It was constructed of a very hard flesh-colored plastic, much more user friendly. But it did not leave any room for my breasts to grow, or give me any kind of shape, which of course are important for a fourteen year old. I wore that brace for about one and a half years. I didn't go back to school until after the mid-year semester break. I tested out again and was able to move on to the ninth grade after only attending four months of eighth grade. Thank God for my intelligence.

The year between thirteen and fourteen years of age was significant: I had major surgeries, the previous year I had been cavity free, but the year of my fusion, I developed fourteen cavities, Charlene died that year, and Mom and Dad divorced. During those many years of marriage, my Dad made a living as a carpenter. He also had alcohol, gambling and womanizing problems. I remember many fond experiences with my Dad previous to polio: picnics, fishing trips, planting flowers, etc. After three of his children came down with polio, he relied more and more on the booze to numb his pain. Unfortunately, our father was mostly absent, either drunk, or just wasn't at home, after we had polio. When he was home, he and Mom fought horribly. Finally, Mom had had enough of the fighting and lack of support. She filed for divorce.

That same year, Dr. Stevenson, at St. Elizabeth's Hospital in Yakima, performed a tendon transplant on my left hand. He attached the tendons from my fourth finger, my strongest finger on that hand, to my thumb muscle. This was to give my thumb the ability to flex outward to give me the opposable action. It didn't work; the finger wasn't strong enough. The following summer of 1959, at age fifteen, the back brace was shed forever. I was BRACE FREE!! I could actually wear summer tops and sandals.

Meanwhile, Mother had miraculously completed two years at the local community college. She now needed to finish her teaching degree at Central Washington State College in Ellensburg, Washington. So the next year, the summer after ninth grade we moved and I attended Ellensburg High School. Since I was starting high school, I wanted to be in the pep band. I had learned how to hold the drumsticks in my left hand so I could perform quite well. I also enjoyed playing the piano; I wasn't that skilled, but I could play a nice melody to accompany singing. However, the doctors had convinced Mom that a "bone block" in my left hand could give me the opposable action, making it possible for me to grip objects. I argued against the operation. "I can balance a glass of water on the back of my hand. I can play the drums and the piano to my satisfaction. I don't need this surgery!" I protested. However, they proceeded. Dr. Nash at children's Hospital, the same surgeon who did the ankle tendon transplant, was going to operate. I went into the procedure knowing they were going to put an extra bone in my hand. They neglected to tell me from where would they get the bone. When I woke up, I was thoroughly surprised that my left leg, my "good" leg, hurt. The "extra" bone's origin was from my left shin bone. Great! they put a scar on my good leg without asking me, I won't be able to play the piano any longer and I can not manipulate the drumsticks well enough to do rolls and such. But I can grip a glass of water now. I was angry. Angry that they had not followed Dr. Lacocq's lead and told me the whole story before surgery. I was angry that they left me out of the loop. It was my body, but no one ever asked me, before or after, how I felt.

However, a few years later when I gripped my baby's diaper with my left hand and pinned it together with my right hand, I thanked Dr. Nash immensely. That operation made it possible for me to grip a steering wheel, braid my daughter's hair, and squeeze my husband's hand. We tend to not think of these basic abilities. Thank you again Dr. Nash. Now that I was brace free, I thought polio was basically over. But I was wrong.

PART III: A DIFFERENT PLAYGROUND

I braced myself for the adult playground with polio residuals: I walked with a decided short-leg limp, I was unable to run, skip, or jump, my left forearm and hand were severely compromised, my right shoulder muscles were very atrophied making it impossible to reach up or out with that arm, my ribcage was rotated making my right shoulder blade protrude; my neck and back were limited in function. But I had weathered it all. I was strong enough to complete a mild-five-mile hike. I went back to playing drums, although with less dexterity. I marched in a parade during my senior year.

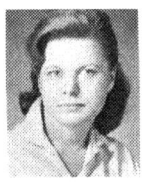

Age 18

I graduated, moved away from home, living in my own apartment. I worked as a waitress in a bowling alley and went to college during the daytime hours. I then applied to Washington State Vocational Rehabilitation to help me finance my college tuition. By the second quarter, they offered me even more than I had expected, so I moved in with four other college girls and quit my waitress job.

At the same time, I met a solider who was TDY (temporary duty) at the Yakima Firing Range, just outside Yakima. I met him the week that President Kennedy was assassinated, November 1963, and by April 4,1964, Hank and I were married. April 13th I turned twenty. One month later we returned to his permanent duty station at Ft. Lewis near Tacoma, Washington. We moved into a little apartment near by and began a normal and traditional married life: I took care of the house and home responsibilities and he earned our living expenses.

Since Hank was a solider, we were stationed in various locations. We weren't even married a year when he received orders for Korea for a 13 month, unaccompanied (meaning that I could not go) tour of duty. During that separation I lived with his mother in Wilkes-Barre, Pennsylvania. After Korea he was stationed in Landstuhl, Germany, this time I could join him after a couple of months.

We lived in government quarters which consisted of at least thirty buildings. Each building was constructed with three stairwells which were three stories high.. Six apartments were in each stairwell making a total of eighteen. The basement included both laundry and storage facilities.

Your laundry days were assigned according to your location. Doing laundry was one of those challenges because of polio. You see I lived on the second floor, so I had to carry my laundry down three flights of stairs and then back up again. The difficulty is that my one leg was very atrophied and I did not have the use of the muscles that would pull my body up the stairs in my right leg. So, I took the stairs one at a time with my left leg only. A few years later when we were stationed in Germany again, I needed to do this with my children who were 3½, 2, and new born. Laundry day was exhausting, but I found a way to do it. It was like polio was playing a game with me, always presenting with a new challenge.

I loved the travel of the military life; I was enthralled with the different cultures. While in Germany the first time, I went exploring and found an old grandfather clock, with all its original parts and glass, laying on the dirt basement floor of a little clock shop. It worked fine; it kept good time. I bought it dirt cheap, $60.00. When I returned to the United States I discovered it was worth $4000. Such adventures were fun.

Polio played hide-n-seek with me; I never knew when it would pop up again. We were only in Germany eight months when he got orders for Viet Nam! It was July 1967 and the "war" was in full swing. Hank being a career solider was proud to serve his country. I stayed home and lived in a little one bedroom house near Yakima Valley College, where I had once attended. One evening, about a month after Hank had departed, terrible abdominal cramps, which I had never previously experienced, wracked my body. The pain bent me over and knocked me off my feet. Dr. Waters, whose name I had randomly drawn from a phone book, called in a prescription for pain relief to the local pharmacy and told me to come to his office in the morning if I still had trouble. After regurgitating the pain medication, and spending a sleepless night of pain, I was one of the first people in line at his office the next morning. The minute I sat down the cramps completely stopped! I decided to stay but I had no further pain. Before sitting in his private office, he had given me a brief pelvic examination. As I sat in a big overstuffed chair, he explained to me that he could find nothing that would cause the cramping. He wanted me to know that, due to me having polio, I "probably cannot have children." I was devastated. At age twenty-three, I had been married three years and desperately wanted a family. He continued telling me, "I am the guardian of a young, under-aged, woman who is giving her baby up for adoption. Would you be interested in adopting?"

This was happening too fast; I was still stuck on his words "probably cannot have children."

After a tearful couple of days, I contacted him once again. After talking it over with Hank (through letters), we proceeded to make arrangements for the adoption. Mr. John Lust, my lawyer, took care of all the legalities. He coordinated everything with the Judge Advocate in Viet Nam. Then we waited for the baby's arrival; she was due mid-November, I had been told. She waited until December 7, 1967. On the ninth I would take her home. However, I received a phone call from Mr. Lust that interrupted the plan. The judge said that before he could declare the adoption final, the prospective father, in Viet Nam, had to be informed of her birth, her gender, and her health. Once the father had signed a declaration of this information, then the judge would finalize the adoption. This was an unexpected turn of events, and Mr. Lust was not available to attend court with me on that final day. So a substitute lawyer from his firm stood beside me at the final decree. On December 11, 1967, Tracy became our daughter. This would not have happened except that polio gave me the message of "probably cannot have children."

I brought our baby home to my little house on Bonnie Doone St. when she was four days old. Tracy was my whole life. I woke when she awakened, ate on her schedule, took naps when she slept, and played, rocked and cooed with her. I loved her completely.

However, when she was five weeks old, I slipped and fell on the ice. My left ankle was broken, that meant that I could not get up because the break was in my "good" leg and my right leg was too weak from polio to lift me off the ground. I sat on the ice and hollered for help, while my baby was in her crib. After a while my neighbor came out and found me. My sister, Thada, was called. At the hospital we discovered it was broken in three places and needed an operation to repair the torn tendons. I could not manage crutches because my right shoulder and left forearm muscles were too compromised. Therefore I needed a wheelchair. Alone I could not care for myself or my baby. I lived with Thada and Art, my sister's husband, for the next five weeks until I could put weight on that ankle.

When Tracy was eight months old, August 1968, Hank came home from Viet Nam. He had made it through the "Tet Offensive" unscathed physically, but he brought home his tortured experiences and "agent orange."

Like all good soldiers, we pushed on to the next tour of duty, Ft. Benning, Georgia. We had a month's leave to get organized and move. Everything was in a transitional state, including my "periods." My monthly menstrual cycle had never been regular and for the past four years I had received a hormone shot every few months to jumpstart my period. When Hank returned from Viet Nam, my periods stopped. So in November, at the OB/GYN clinic at Martin Army Hospital, Ft. Benning, Georgia, I expected receiving my standard pelvic exam and hormone shot. Instead the doctor said I was about three months pregnant. I was stunned and then overjoyed. Scott was born by natural birth on May 14, 1969. I had a long and difficult delivery because I didn't have the muscle strength to push him through the birth canal, a polio residual. This is probably what Dr. Waters had been talking about, problems with delivery, not conception.   However, I believe he had been vague because he was looking for parents for Tracy. That worked out fine for Hank, Tracy and I.

Scott was a joyful gift, for sure. He was only about two months old, when "Daddy Soldier" was sent off again. This time back to Germany. The children and I waited at his Mother's house in Wilkes-Barre, Pennsylvania. About six months later, 8 days before departure, we received a notice for a flight out of Kennedy International Airport for Frankfurt, Germany. He was stationed at a base near Stuttgart. We again lived in a government housing complex named Pattonville.

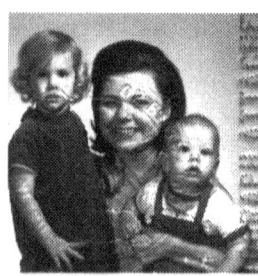

Passport Picture, age 2, 25, 9 months

We arrived in Germany in February. Settled in for our three year tour when on May 7th, Hank, whose 36th birthday was in April, had a massive heart attack that put him in the hospital for about a month. The following convalescent leave was for six months.

Here I was in a foreign country, speaking no German, with no personal support system. At that time phone calls to home were out of the question because of their high cost. My family of origin was not an emotionally supportive family. Tracy was 2½, Scott turned one while Hank was in the hospital, and by July, I was pregnant with Marla. She was born on April 22, 1971. Three children, all under 4 years old. That tour was quite an adventure.

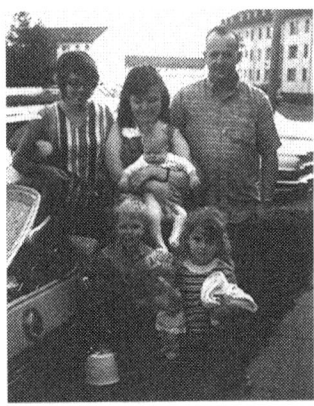

Rhonda, Val, Hank, Marla (in my arms) Scotty and Tracy.
You can see one of the American Pattonville housing buildings in the background.

Although my children were very close in age, I loved being their Mommie. Apart from idiotic comments, biases, and prejudices, I continued my life quite joyfully within the limitations of my disabilities.

The German wife who lived across the hall in my stairwell, told me that the reason you don't see disabled people on the streets in Germany, was because the German people sent their "defective people" away to live in institutions so the rest of the public "don't have to look at them." She was totally serious, and very wrong. Another neighbor, also a German wife of an American solider, told me that my husband took me as his second wife (it was true that Hank had been married before) because he knew that I would not cheat on him. She said he knew I would be so grateful to him because of my handicap. Since she was also the second wife of her husband, I wanted to ask her if her handicap was mental. But I was still shy enough to not say it.

So polio was a slow merry-go-round in my everyday life. My residuals remained fairly stable during these years. I was limited from many activities because of the effects of polio, but I did most everything I wanted. Hank's last tour of duty was Ft. Carson at Colorado Springs, Colorado. As I was growing mentally and emotionally, my marriage was failing. In 1976, I started back to school. Vocational Rehabilitation helped me financially with the first two years of my education. At first I wanted to just expand myself, learning more both internally and externally. In '77 Hank and I separated briefly, which motivated me to look at how I could make a living if we did split up.

In April 1978, Hank and I tried a geographical cure; we moved to a small mountain town at the base of Pikes Peak, Woodland Park, CO. October we legally separated and the marriage was over. My disabilities limited my vocational possibilities, I couldn't stand for long periods of time, I was unable to type well enough for a job, I can not raise my right arm above my head, my left hand did not have adequate dexterity. I needed more education. With Vocational Rehabilitation's financial aid, academic scholarships, and government grants and loans, I completed the work for my Bachelor of Arts in Counseling Psychology. I worked as a crisis, residential, and rehabilitation counselor to help support my children while I attended school. Hank did pay child support sporadically. I was proud that I never received public financial assistance. I believed that God loved me and I was going to be a therapist one day.

I had become quite comfortable and complacent about my disabilities. However, polio began playing with me again in about 1980. First I had to have my prolapsed uterus removed. I was told that due to weakened muscles, my uterus had dropped, and created a herniated bladder, therefore a partial hysterectomy was needed. Polio just kept showing its ugly face.

In '81-'83 I attended classes at the University of Colorado at Colorado Springs (UCCS). Because the campus was built on a hill, I became increasingly fatigued while walking from class to class. I couldn't get my breath and would get dizzy and light-headed, just walking. I made it though. I received my BA in May, 1983 and moved with my two girls and my boyfriend of two years, Rob, into a new residence. Scott, my son lived with his father, Hank. The day after we moved, Hank was hospitalized for chest pain. Two days later he experienced a massive heart attack which resulted in brain death. He was a vegetable. They had brought his heart back, but his brain went 45 minutes without oxygen. Six days later, on June 22, 1983, Hank was dead.

I was so tired and discouraged, I didn't feel like I could continue my hectic life. I had three teenage children who were acting out all their anger, a new relationship, a full time job, and I needed to further my education so I could work less manual jobs. My goal was to become a mental health therapist.

Rob was so supportive through all this. He was a perfect step-father, who waited in the sidelines, never bossing or taking over. We loved each other dearly. In November 1984, Rob and I wed while my three children stood as witnesses.

I left my full-time position and took a part time job as a ward clerk in the psychiatric ward of St. Francis Hospital.. I had only been there about six weeks when I sprained my left ankle, my good leg again. I seemed to be getting weaker and falling down more often. Because my leg was in a non-weight-bearing cast, I wasn't able to continue my job. Shortly after that I was offered a position as a rehabilitation counselor, which I took once my foot healed. I also started a weekend program for a Master's Degree.

By 1985, Polio was once again making its reality more and more apparent in my life. I was still working towards my master's degree and was scheduled to speak to the high school psychology classes about the holidays and depression. Colorado can have some nasty cold weather. This particular day I was walking across the outdoor commons at Coronado High School in a mild blizzard. My legs just QUIT! I could not make my left leg, my good leg, move. It was like I was frozen to that spot. The young man, who was my guide, just looked at me as if I was crazy. We stood still in this blizzard for a couple of minutes and then the messages to my muscles kicked in and I was able to walk once again. Now I am actually shaking from both the cold and my own fear. I was able to give a successful presentation. That was the first symptom of what the medical community has named Post Polio Syndrome.

By January of 1987, I had finished my Education and started teaching undergraduate courses in psychology in the evenings and working full time for Rocky Mountain Rehabilitation Center as a psychotherapist. One of my duties was to manage the Post Polio Clinic. Post Polio Syndrome is a group of symptoms that up to 50% of polio survivors experience

20-40- years after the initial illness. Those nerve horn cells that the virus first attacked die off faster than the same cells die in a non-afflicted person. Since I was substantially paralyzed initially, a huge number of my cells had been compromised, either damaged or dead.

The walk from the parking lot to my classroom, where I taught courses at Pikes Peak Community College, was becoming nearly impossible. I sought advice from my doctor because my left arm ached and sometimes my chest hurt. He thought it might be my heart too, so he ordered various tests. My heart was strong but it was complaining. A sleep study was conducted and it was discovered that my nocturnal blood oxygen content dropped to a low of 49%. That is exceptionally low; the average is 93%-99%. So I was probably not getting enough oxygen to my heart at other times. The primary doctor and the pulmonary specialist decided if I had better sleep (with more oxygen) my body would function better during the day. I began using nocturnal oxygen assistance in 1989. I was very discouraged at first and I almost hated the machinery. However, I developed a relationship with my oxygen concentrator; I talked with it like I would a co-worker that I needed to learn to accept. I grew to love my concentrator. Two years passed again and my muscles were continuing to weaken. Again I experienced overwhelming fatigue, headache and weakness. It was in February of 1991 that my doctors were talking about conducting a tracheotomy and putting me on a ventilator. Since I was working in a pain clinic, I asked a few other doctors their opinions. Several of them said I could possibly breathe easier if I were at a lower elevation.

During spring break, Rob and I visited Chico, California and Medford, Oregon, two places where there were possible job leads in his field of wholesale plumbing. We went back home and thought it over. Even though we had no jobs, no family with us, one set of friends who lived on Table Rock Road, and a small savings account, in June 1991, Rob and I took a huge risk. We packed up and moved to Medford, Oregon, polio's new playground for us. All of my adult children decided to stay in Colorado (Marla was the youngest at age 19.) Rob's one daughter, Alison, age 13 still lived with her mother in Aurora, Colorado.

We truly missed our family and also loved being in Oregon. We both found good jobs in our fields of expertise by the end of three months. In my opinion, my breathing and muscle strength were so much better I didn't even go see a doctor for seven months. (March 10, 1992 my granddaughter, Samantha was born.) When I did see Dr. Eric Overland in 1992, he put me on a recently developed bi-pap (bilateral positive air pressure) machine to further assist my nighttime breathing.. It is a great invention; it basically breathes for me while I sleep, sucking the air in and pushing it out.

With valuable sleep returned to me, I now loved both my concentrator and my bi-pap machine. However, the rest of my body was losing function too. I was becoming more and more fatigued. I was falling down on an average of every two weeks. My right leg would just collapse on me. I quit all shopping, including grocery shopping, and we did not go on any vacations for two years because I just couldn't walk enough to enjoy it. I was terribly fatigued. Rob, with never a derisive word, picked up the slack for all those undone domestic chores.

After seeing a physiatrist, I began using a motorized wheelchair in 1994. At first I was quite devastated; it felt like all my effort to learn to walk again was now failing. I thought it was the lowest dip of polio's roller coaster ride. What I soon discovered was that the wheelchair actually gave me more freedom because I was once again mobile. I could even enjoy shopping once again, as well as, trips to the park when my family came to see me. (My grandson, Riley, was born October 1994.)

From early 1994--1999, I worked for the Medford, Oregon's Children's Advocacy Center where I specialized in the treatment of abused children, mostly sex abuse. I became an expert in the field, reading voraciously, attending educational conferences, workshops, seminars and college classes. I often testified in court, and gave special training workshops, which I still conduct. In 1997, as a part of a team of experts, I was invited to present at a Washington DC summit for the National Justice Programs in Washington D.C. Our team consisted of a Jackson County Court Judge,

Mark Schively, the Jackson County District Attorney, Mark Huddleson, a polygraph expert, Susan Holmes, a probation/parole officer, Sam Olsen, a sex offender therapist, David Robinson, and me, as a victim therapist. The purpose of this summit was to decide how to best use a two million dollar allotment to manage sex offenders in our communities. Jackson County, Oregon was chosen as a national model because of a study which indicated we had a 1% recidivism rate of offenders who had completed our treatment program. Out of this summit the "Center for Sex Offender Management" (CSOM) was created.

The National Justice Programs flew us to Washington DC, housed us at the Renaissance Hotel, where they hold regal dinners and/or other entertainment for dignitaries or heads of foreign countries. I felt so privileged and rewarded for all my hard career work.

On the airplane, I had to carry with me my wheelchair, a wheelchair charger, an oxygen concentrator, my bi-pap machine, and my regular luggage. The oxygen concentrator was about 18" wide by 24" deep and 36" high. It pulled the air in, through a filter, and pumped out 95-99% oxygen. Tubing from the concentrator attaches to the bi-pap machine, which was about 12" long, 6" high, and about 8" wide. The bi-pap forced the oxygenated air into my lungs and then pulled my expiration out of my lungs. The muscles that operate my lungs had become too weak to do this for myself when I sleep. Attached to the bi-pap was a large hose which ended in a face mask. This mask, held on by a conglomeration of straps (head gear), covered my nose and sealed a vacuum around my nose and upper lip. The wheelchair charger was about 12 x 12 x 12 inches and quite heavy.

Everything but the luggage had to be carried right with me because I could not breathe without my machines. My traveling companions and I operated as a team; they received special treatment at the boarding counter because they were with a disabled person, and I received their assistance in carrying this equipment. Mark Huddleson pushed my concentrator along, while Judge Shively, Sam Olsen, and David Robinson took turns toting the bi-pap and the charger. This little country girl traveling to Washington DC as part of a team of experts, felt pretty high on polio's teeter-totter.

In 1999, my lack of oxygen in my system and the stressful child abuse cases made it necessary for me to leave the Children's Advocacy Center. Then I took a position as Directors of Crisis and Treatment Services at Community Works where I directed and managed 8 programs. I had to finally admit that I could no longer maintain the amount of physical energy it took to continue with that kind of workload. I left that position after only one year to reduce my workload.

By now, I was using the wheelchair everywhere but in my office and at home. The weakness in my body was increasing, especially my hips and my lungs. But I loved my career and my work, so my next adventure was working 25 hours per week as a counselor for troubled kids at McLoughlin Middle School and continuing my private practice for a few hours a week. However, I closed my private practice in 2002. Now I needed oxygen assist 24/7. I had to start carrying a Helios Oxygen unit for my waking hours. I resigned the middle school position in June 2003.

The Helios system holds liquid oxygen that is pushed into my lungs. I even have to shower with it. My pulmonary specialist, Dr. Overland, tells me that my lungs are only operating at 40% of that of an average woman my age. I will probably need a ventilator in the future, maybe the near future, maybe not. But my next chosen career, writing, can be done from home at my pace. There is nothing that can stop the decrease of those nerve cells so I have to make the most of what have. I want to make the most of my time. This polio ride can be exhausting.

Although I still use the bi-pap, oxygen concentrator, Helios unit, and my wheelchair, I am very active in volunteer work, spiritual gatherings and writing. A few months ago, Dr. O'Sullivan, a neck and spine specialist, said I have the neck of a ninety year old. But I've adapted to this Polio playground this far. I do get discouraged at times, but there are still adventures waiting for me; motorized wheelchair adventures at six miles per hour. Some of these experiences happen while traveling the Bear Creek Greenway Bike Path. Some of them happen while traveling the streets and roadways between Central Point and Medford, Oregon. Some of them happen in stores or at church. These adventures are fascinating and make life wonderful.

I want to leave you with a couple of thoughts. I have worked to make my life fulfilling in the richest country in the world and no matter where the playground took me. What would my life have been in a country where Polio is still running amok: India, Nigeria, Pakistan, Egypt, Afghanistan, Niger, and Somalia (listed from highest to lowest burden of disease). 99% of the cases are in India, Nigeria, and Pakistan. Also, there are six other countries considered at high risk for re-infection of poliomyelitis: Angola, Bangladesh, Dominican Republic of the Congo, Ethiopia, Nepal, and Sudan. The new cases reported by the World Health Organization (WHO) on May 20, 2004 are as follows: Nigeria (133), Niger, (12), Pakistan (12), India (8), Afghanistan (2), Egypt (2), and Somalia(0). On January 15, 2004 "The Geneva Declaration for the Eradication of Poliomyelitis" was pronounced by Dr. Lee Jong-wook, WHO Director-General. All seven countries' heads of state signed also. President Bush has declared 2004 as the "Year of Polio Eradication." (Information paraphrased from "Post-Polio Health International Annual Report.")

If I was in one of these countries, I would not have lived. I would not have been able to contribute to my community, not have been able to counsel those people I have helped successfully, I would not have been a contributor to the National Center for Sex Offender Management. And, I would not have been able to ask you to contribute whatever you possibly can to eradicate polio throughout the world. Please, give your services, educate when you can, give financial contributions, whatever is possible to stop the pain of this devastating disease.

In conclusion, there is one thing of which I am sure; I am perfect as I am. I am a vessel for human compassion. I bring out the goodness in others. I enjoy life and people see that I am happy. My life with polio has been a roller coaster ride bringing me wonderful people and opportunities, my daughter Tracy, my education/career. And polio has taught me very useful life lessons, endurance and courage. My soul and my spirit have been enriched by these people and experiences. I love the freedom of my wheelchair and the life affirmation of my oxygen machines. I am blessed.

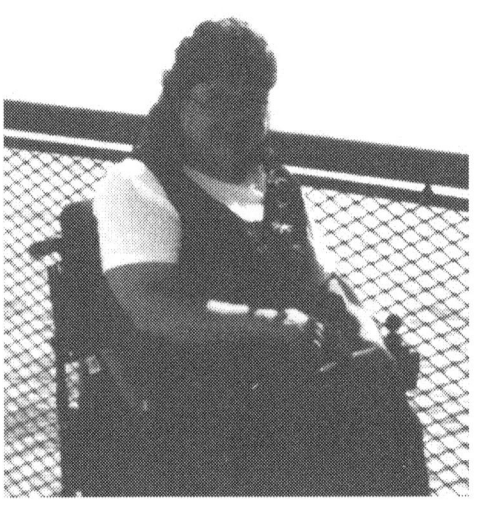

Epilogue

—

Since this is the second edition publication, in late 2005, here is a little update. I'm still breathing without a tracheotomy or a ventilator. My lung capacity has not decreased!! Yeah!! My spirit is as strong or stronger than ever. And I am near completion on a creative non-fiction novel tentatively titled "The Gift of Obstacles."

I have three grandchildren and two great grand children. Marla and her husband, Tony, moved out to Oregon to be close. I'm getting a little weaker in my muscles each year. But I am enjoying life as much as ever.

Unfortunately, polio has not been completely eradicated throughout the world. However, we have made more progress and continue to work with countries who are resistant due to political ideologies. I hope that polio will soon follow the path of Latin; it will become the dead language of disease, especially with your ongoing contributions. Thank-you.

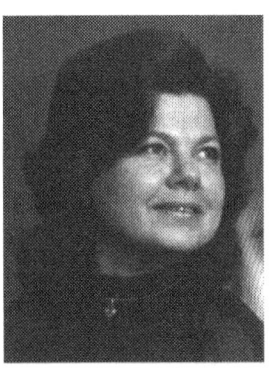

About the Author

Valerie J. Foster is a poet and writer who retired from a 25-year-career in mental health counseling, specializing in child sex abuse recovery, and is now devoting more time to the art of writing. Her poetry is published in two anthologies of poetry, "Chorus of the Soul," (International Poetry, 2000) and "Invoking the Muse" (International Poetry, February 2005) Valerie's other works have received local publication. Her original memoir "My Life with Polio" was published in November 2004 by Jmar Publications. Valerie grew up in Yakima, Washington where she and her two older sisters met the challenge of poliomyelitis. Although left with deforming residuals, later, she married a solider, raised their three children as they traveled across the United States and in Europe. Now, she and her current husband live in Central Point, Oregon. Valerie is working on a book tentatively titled "The Gift of Obstacles," about meeting the challenges of life: poverty, abuse, death, divorce, promiscuity, depression, suicide, education, and employment.